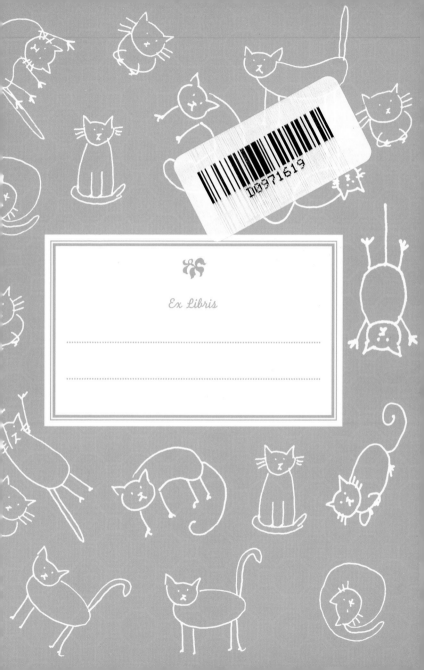

Ex Libris

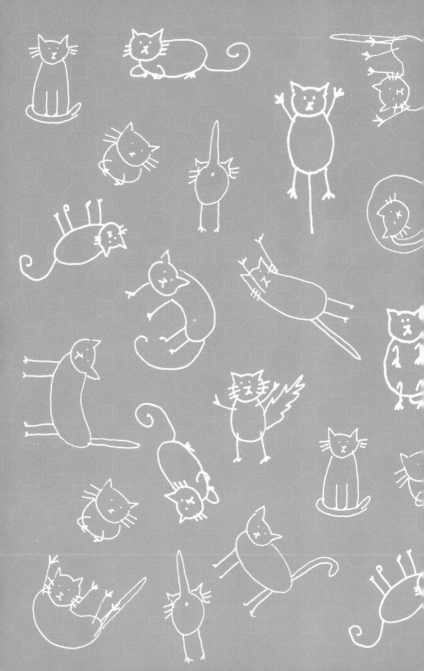

YOGA FOR CATS

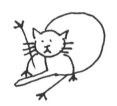

First published in the United States of America in 2004
by UNIVERSE PUBLISHING
A Division of Rizzoli International Publications, Inc.
300 Park Avenue South
New York, NY 10010
www.rizzoliusa.com

Text © 2003 by Christiénne Wadsworth
Illustrations and photographs © 2003 by Lynn Chang-Franklin

2004 2005 2006 2007/ 10 9 8 7 6 5 4 3 2 1

Distributed in the U.S. trade by St. Martin's Press, New York

Printed in Mexico

ISBN: 0-7893-1080-5

Library of Congress Control Number: 2004103106

Designed by Lynn Chang-Franklin

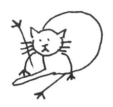

YOGA FOR CATS

By Christiénne Wadsworth
Illustrated by Lynn Chang-Franklin

Universe

TABLE OF CONTENTS

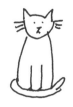

Not sure if Yoga is for you?
Try the Yoga Quiz, pages 2–3.

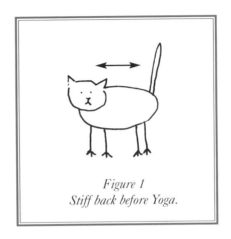

Figure 1
Stiff back before Yoga.

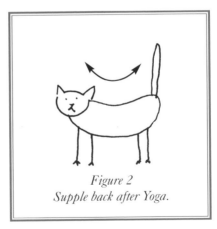

Figure 2
Supple back after Yoga.

INTRODUCTION

*D*ear Reader, Are you edgy, jumpy and wary? Are you overweight and is your overall appearance best described as slovenly? If so, this book is for you. Full of time-honored poses such as *Cinnashta* (The Cinnamon Bun), *Thanksalotta* (The Turkey), and *Freakedoutunda* (The Warrior), this easy-to-use guide will help you reap the benefits of the ancient practice of Yoga, step by step.

By working lovingly on a Yoga practice, you will find that like your ancestors, you will soon be able to defy gravity, appear to have no skeletal structure, and manage to sleep in the most impossible places for hours.

Read on, my friend. You'll find the following pages will not only enlighten human companions everywhere, but will also provide harmony and understanding in homes where felines and humans meet.

Namaste.

Christiénne Wadsworth
Los Angeles
November 2003

The Yoga Quiz

This quiz will help you determine whether Yoga is for you.

1. The usual position for your feet is:

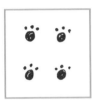 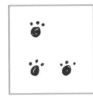 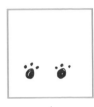

a.   b.   c.   d.

2. I find that my ability to spring easily from a sitting position on the floor up onto the bed is:

a. no challenge at all.
b. slight challenge.
c. increasingly difficult.
d. completely inhibited by my swinging belly skin.

3. The shape of my body most resembles:

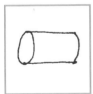

a.   b.   c.   d.
a tube.   an almond. a pear.   a cheese wheel.

Do you spend an inordinate amount of time obsessing over a nonexistent spot on the wall?

a.   No, I spend my time philosophizing.
b.   Sometimes.
c.   Wait, there *is* a spot on the wall?
d.   A great deal of time.

My fitness routine consists of:

a.   waking up slowly, followed by an all-body stretch, a small breakfast, and racing and leaping around the house and yard.
b.   racing and leaping around the house and yard.
c.   racing around the house.
d.   waking the humans to feed me, grazing, finding a sunny spot, and going back to sleep.

My typical diet consists of:

a.   a soy bean–based dry cat food and mountain-spring bottled water.
b.   dry but tasty cat food and water.
c.   wet cat food three times a day at specified hours. (Only my favorite brand or I throw up a hair ball on the newly dry-cleaned bed coverlet.)
d.   wet cat food. Dog's food in dish. Lint and holiday tinsel left underneath couch, topped with fried chicken leg stolen from kitchen table.

f you answered a. to most questions, then you can benefit from the xpert Yoga tips in this book. If you answered b., c., or d., then you are typical cat and desperately need Yoga in your life.

ather than meow about it, or procrastinate by staring at the dripping faucet, use the following tips to help you make the leap into your practice.

When:

It's important to start a routine. For example, a good time might be when you get up at 3 a.m. and want to be fed.

Duration:

Being a feline is a time-consuming job, but it's important to squeeze in some time for Yoga.

Setting:

Find your special spot. The best ones are usually where you are not allowed: on the bed, on the sofa, in the sunbeam on the table, etc.

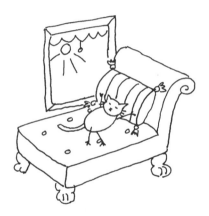

*C*hakras are subtle, dynamic vortexes that are important to your body, like your paws or your tail, as well as to your Cat Yoga practice.

Energy, also known as prana, flows through these chakras. The energy is like the electricity you can't see but whose effect you experience when you bite into that lamp cord.

The chart at the right demonstrates the location of your chakras, and where to lick when you're feeling one of them may be blocked.

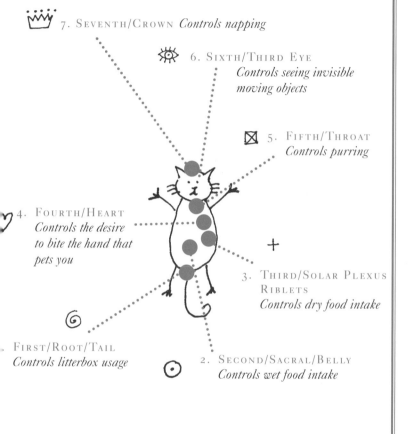

7. SEVENTH/CROWN *Controls napping*

6. SIXTH/THIRD EYE
Controls seeing invisible moving objects

5. FIFTH/THROAT
Controls purring

4. FOURTH/HEART
Controls the desire to bite the hand that pets you

3. THIRD/SOLAR PLEXUS RIBLETS
Controls dry food intake

FIRST/ROOT/TAIL
Controls litterbox usage

2. SECOND/SACRAL/BELLY
Controls wet food intake

Feline Chakras.

PURRING

*P*urring not only releases tension, it also allows you to escape into a world where every dish is filled with fresh tuna fish, and every bed, couch, and chair is soft, snuggly, void of any dog slobber, and only for you.

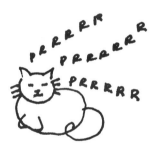

Purring in semi "Pain au Chocolat" pose.
See pages 32–33.

VOCALIZATIONS

ou'll find many Yoga Masters will utilize vocalizations during their practice. Whether you use yowls to dispel negative energy at the beginning or even a combination of purrs and mews while holding a pose, developing your own sound repetoire will add richness to your practice.

SOME SUGGESTED VOCALIZATIONS:

Maaaaaaa

Maaaa Maaaa

Marrrrhhhhhhh

Meh

Mew

Mew Mew Mew Mew

Meow

Mmmmmmm

MyrrrrOW!

MyrrrrOW?

WARMING UP

*I*t is always important to warm up prior to any exercise. Yoga is no exception. For the outdoor cat, we recommend a light jog around your home. For indoor cats, consider some of our favorite aerobic activities as shown below.

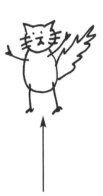

Figure A
Finding balance.

Figure B
Jumping.

THE JUMP.
Simply center yourself on all four feet (Figure A), think of something spooky, and jump as high as you can (Figure B). Fluffing your tail helps with this aerobic exercise.

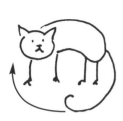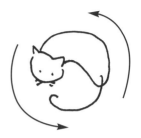

Side View.
Curling tail toward nose.

Top View.
Arrows indicate motion.

CHASING YOUR TAIL.
Center yourself on all four feet, curving your body around an imaginary post or leg. Curl tail toward your nose, then move all four feet forward in synchronized fashion.

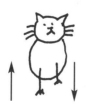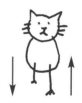

KNEADING.
A low-impact method of getting that circulation flowing.

THE BASICS

*Y*ou will find Cat Yoga will always begin with a few basics, all of which are important to master for a fulfilling and successful Cat Yoga practice.

TOES.
*Release tension in your toes by opening
and closing them as shown.
Toes Closed (left), Toes Spread Wide (right).*

TAIL MUSCLES.
*To begin moving the prana in your tail,
try a series of tail positions as shown.
From left to right: Straight Up, Fluffed Out,
Hooked Right, Hooked Left.*

EYES.
Opening and closing your eyes slowly and rhythmically has a relaxing effect on the entire body.

BREATHING.
Breathing releases tension with the added benefit of cooling your body.
Closing your eyes may help you maximize the benefit of this subtle movement.

POSES

*T*hese positions can be used as a preparation for the standing positions you will find in this guide, but they are also positions in their own right.

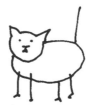

BASIC STANDING POSITION OR
THE MOUNTAIN POSE.
*This classic pose is shown with the tail
in an upright position. To keep this pose steady,
we suggest that you focus your eyes on an
imaginary spot on the wall.*

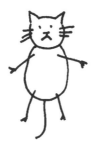

THE CORPSE.
*Lie on back with arms and legs to side.
You may also close your eyes.*

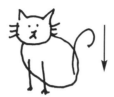

BASIC SITTING POSITION.
*Simply lower your root chakra from
the Basic Standing Position.*

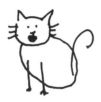

THE LION.
*This pose is the Basic Sitting Position with the
mouth stretched wide into a yawn.*

THE BUG

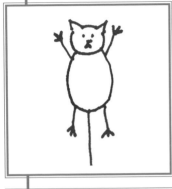

Step 1
Begin on your back and stretch.

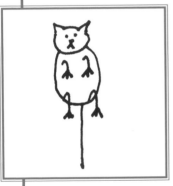

Step 2
Release tension in paws and allow them to curl into a natural position.

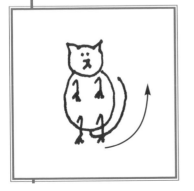

Step 3
Wrap your tail to the right (or left) side of your body.

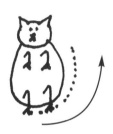

TAILLESS CAT/MANX.
*Wrap your imaginary tail energy to
your side.*

THE CAT

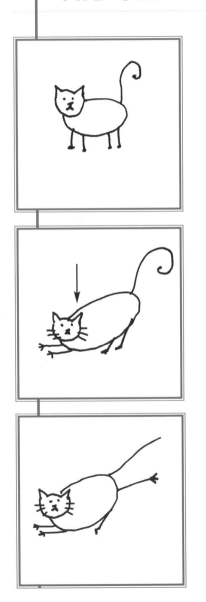

Step 1
Begin in a standing position.

Step 2
Press your chest against the ground, keeping your paws straight in front.

Step 3
Stretch out one leg, as far as it can go, and spread toes. Repeat with other leg.

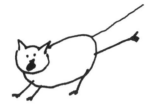

The Cat with a yawn.

THE CINNAMON BUN

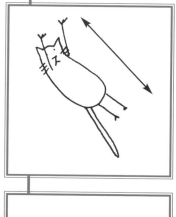

Step 1
Begin in a lying position. Stretch your front paws over your head.

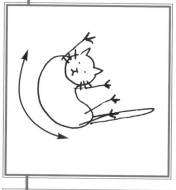

Step 2
Continuing to face the ceiling, curve your back and form a bun position.

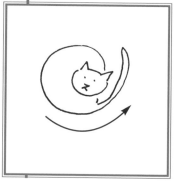

Step 3
Tuck your tail around your body as you continue to face the ceiling.

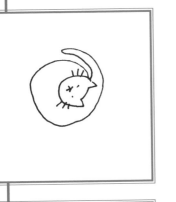

Step 4

Heart, root, and tail chakras meet in this classic bun position.

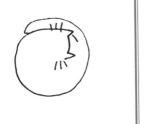

Adjustment.

Turn your face downward and tuck it snugly into your root chakra as shown.

Note: This wonderful position can be held for many, many hours.

CROUCHING TIGER

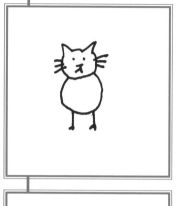

Step 1
Begin in the standing position with pricked ears.

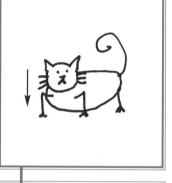

Step 2
Lower your heart chakra to the ground without allowing your belly to touch the ground.

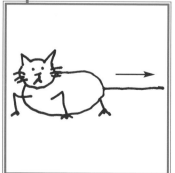

Step 3
Straighten tail behind your body so it is aligned with your spine.

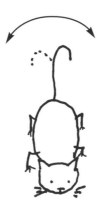

ADJUSTMENT.
Flick tail.

THE FISH HOOK

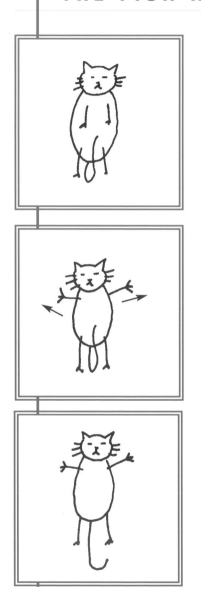

STEP 1

Start on your back with front paws folded and eyes closed tightly.

STEP 2

Extend your front paws out.

STEP 3

Straighten tail and curl to the left or right.

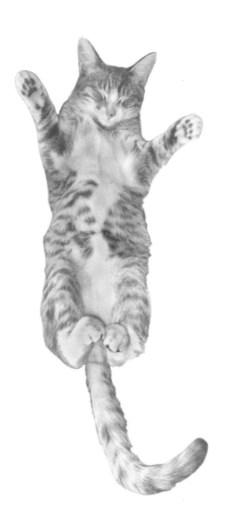

William in the Fish Hook pose

HIDDEN DRAGON

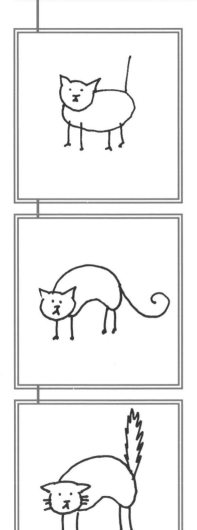

Step 1
Start in a basic standing position.

Step 2
Arch your back, while balanced on all four legs.

Step 3
Flatten ears, fluff tail and raise it straight toward the ceiling, then balance on your tippy toes.

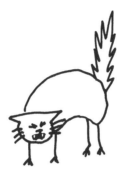

ADJUSTMENT.
Squeeze eyes closed, show fangs, and make frightful sounds.

LONDON BRIDGE

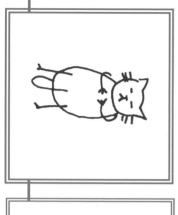

Step 1

Start in a recumbent position with eyes closed tightly.

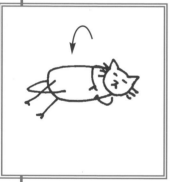

Step 2

Push over to your side.

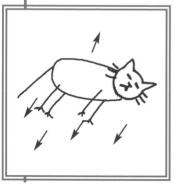

Step 3

Straighten your legs while pushing back in the opposite direction.

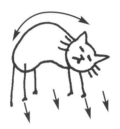

THE LONDON BRIDGE.
*Note the elegant curve of
the back.*

THE MEATLOAF

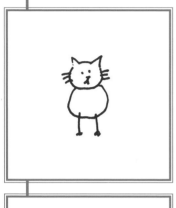

STEP 1
Start in a standing position.

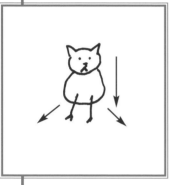

STEP 2
Lower yourself to the ground,
keeping front paws forward.

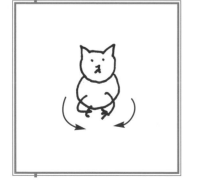

STEP 3
Tuck paws underneath chest so the
paws cannot be seen.

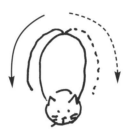

STEP 4
TOP VIEW.
Tuck tail close to body.

PAIN AU CHOCOLAT

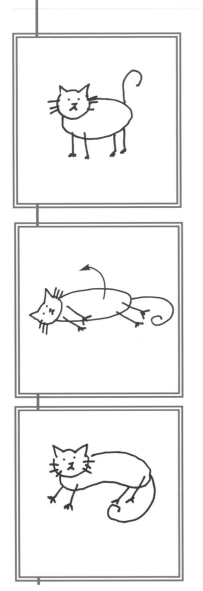

STEP 1

Start in a standing position.

STEP 2

Lightly fall to one side, maintaining head in an upright position.

STEP 3

Arch back slightly and curl tail around front to form the classic *pain au chocolat* shape.

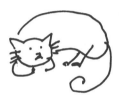

ADJUSTMENT.
*Lower head to floor. This version is often
called The Croissant.*

THE PLANK

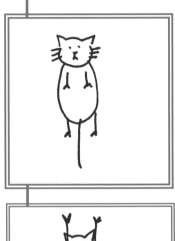

Step 1

Start in a lying position.

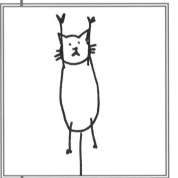

Step 2

Raise paws over head and straighten tail.

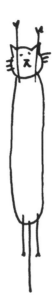

STEP 3

*Continue to stretch your body, imagining that it is made
of taffy and can reach extraordinary lengths. When you
have lengthened your body as much as possible, close your
eyes and hold the position.*

THE SEAL

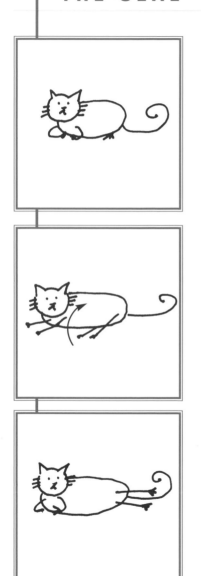

STEP 1
Start in a lying position.

STEP 2
Gently roll onto your side.

STEP 3
Stretch your back legs straight out
from your body, keeping them
touching.

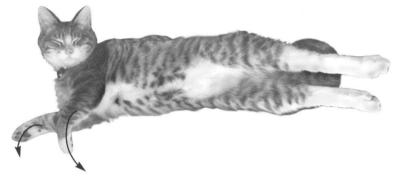

STEP 4
Curl your paws as shown.

THE SPHINX

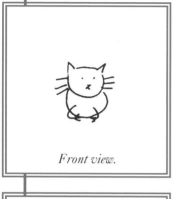

Front view.

STEP 1

Start in a standing position and lower yourself gently to the ground.

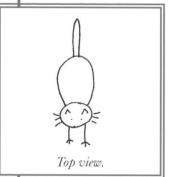

Top view.

STEP 2

Stretch paws in front of yourself while straightening tail so that it aligns with your spine.
Hold position.

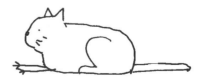

The Sphinx in profile.

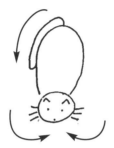

THE SPHINX TRANSFORMING INTO THE
MEATLOAF.
By tucking the tail around the body and the feet.
The Sphinx easily moves into the Meatloaf pose.
See The Meatloaf, pages 30–31.

THE TEAPOT

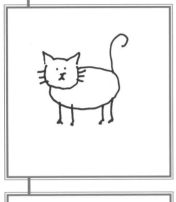

STEP 1

Start in a standing position.

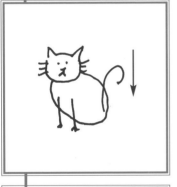

STEP 2

Lower your root chakra to the ground.

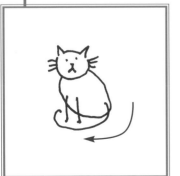

STEP 3

Curl your tail around your paws.

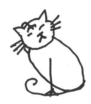

ADJUSTMENT.
Raise right paw and tuck behind right ear.
Repeat with left paw. This is known as
Herbal Tea with Lemon Please.

THE TURKEY

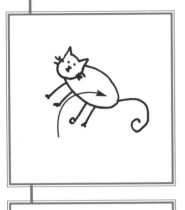

STEP 1
Start in a standing position and fall onto one side.

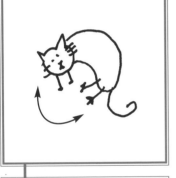

STEP 2
Curl your root chakra to your crown chakra, keeping head slightly raised.

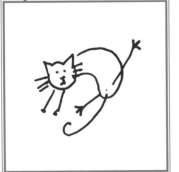

STEP 3
Stretch left leg upward and straddle right leg with front paws.

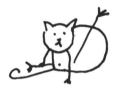

STEP 4
Stretch toes.

THE TWIST

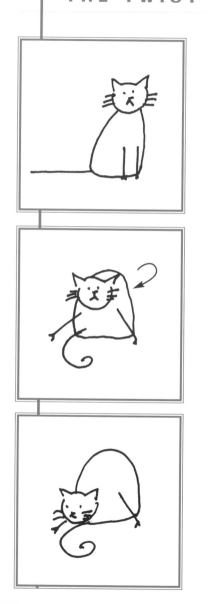

STEP 1
Start in a sitting position.

STEP 2
Maintaining the position of your hind feet and left front paw, twist your upper body and straddle your tail with your right paw.

STEP 3
Lower head toward tail.

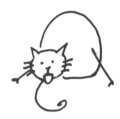

ADJUSTMENT.
Touch your tail with your tongue.

THE VULTURE

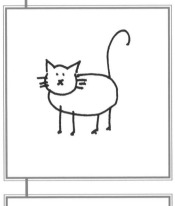

STEP 1
Start in a standing position.

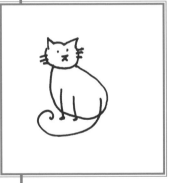

STEP 2
Move gracefully into a sitting position, tucking tail tightly against the body.

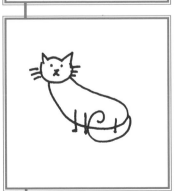

STEP 3
Looking forward, stretch neck and head as far as you can without moving feet.

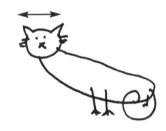

ADJUSTMENTS.
Move head rapidly from side to side,
facing right and then facing left.

THE WARRIOR

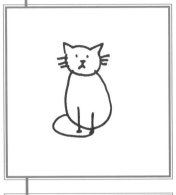

STEP 1
Start in a sitting position.

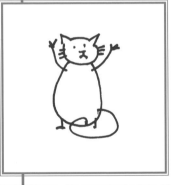

STEP 2
Balance on your root chakra while raising front paws.

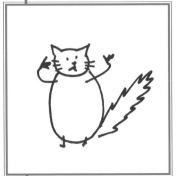

STEP 3
Fluff tail while curving paws and spreading toes.

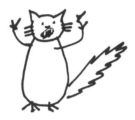

STEP 4

*Open mouth as wide as you can and
emit a piercing scream.*

ADJUSTMENTS

Sometimes when trying to achieve the perfect position, you may want to seek a human hand. Do not feel embarrassed. The following is a demonstration of human adjustment of *Beetleudra, The Bug* position.

Not understanding the beauty and simplicity of *The Bug*, William initially insisted on curving his body while on his back (Figure A and Step 1).

William's human companion then gently rolled William onto his side, pulling slightly and arching his body (Step 2). This allowed William to straighten his back substantially.

Finally, in Step 3, you can see that a gentle push on the exhale enabled William to tilt his chin backward and fully align his chakra flow.

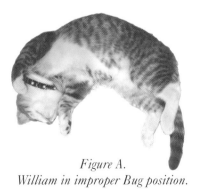

Figure A.
William in improper Bug position.

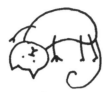

STEP 1
Improper Bug position schematic.

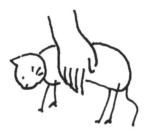

STEP 2
Improving arch.

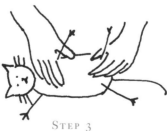

STEP 3
Shift to proper orientation.

CATNIP & YOGA

*C*atnip or "nip," as it is also called, is not recommended for Yog

Please remember catnip is a stimulant, and while the use of catnip heighte aerobic activity—such as leaping from the windowsill to the mantel to th chair to the curtains—it has a negative effect on Yoga.

We strongly suggest you avoid catnip in all forms (balls, mice, powder, mats, etc.) while practicing Yoga.